Claire is Special: Workbook Edition
By Michael R. Basso & Dorothy Scarfone

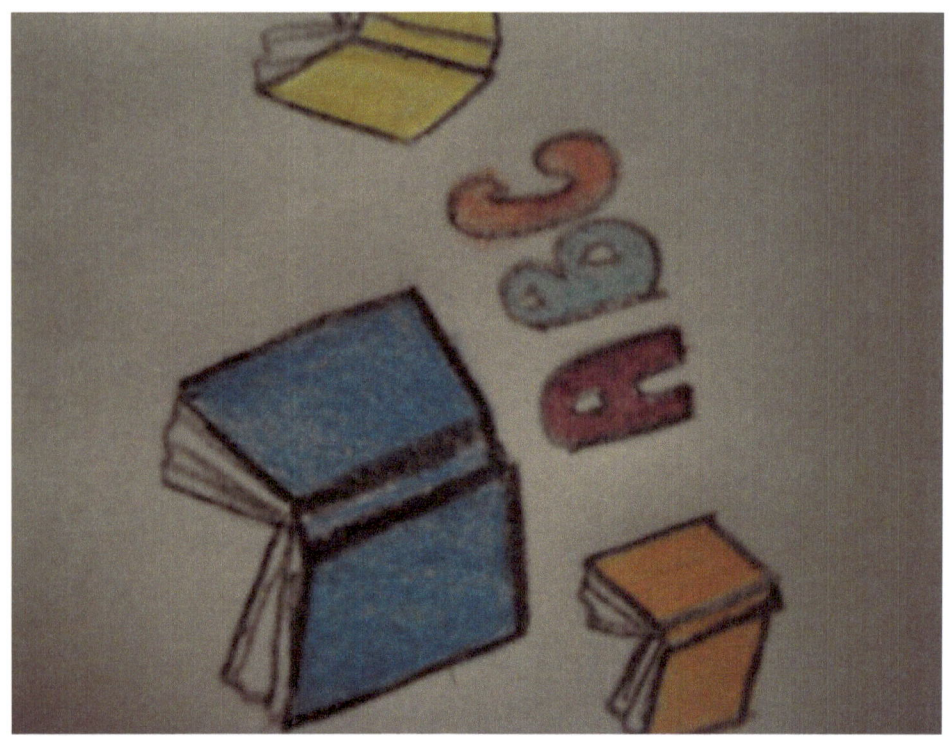

Copyright©2011 by Michael R. Basso and Dorothy Scarfone
ISBN 978-1453857090

Illustrated by Nikki Reyes

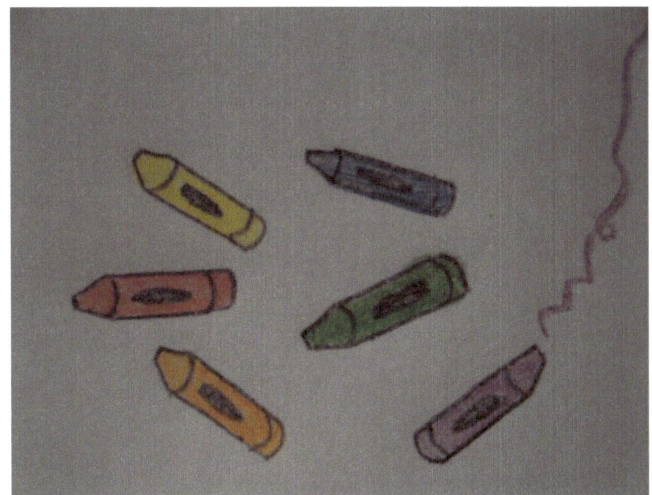

Preface

This is a book for special people and their families. People with Down Syndrome are unique in many ways; some of which can be a challenge for their parents and especially their siblings.

The purpose of this book is to help children learn about the special needs and concerns that their special brothers and sisters have and how the whole family may learn to better cope with the challenges.

Children and adults with Down Syndrome can also be uniquely different in some ways that make them especially loving and dedicated family members. This book is also meant to reinforce those aspects of their being.

A bio.psycho.social approach will be used throughout the book, with due consideration for multicultural diversity and individual differences. Concepts from clinical, social, and developmental psychology and neurobiology will be integrated throughout.

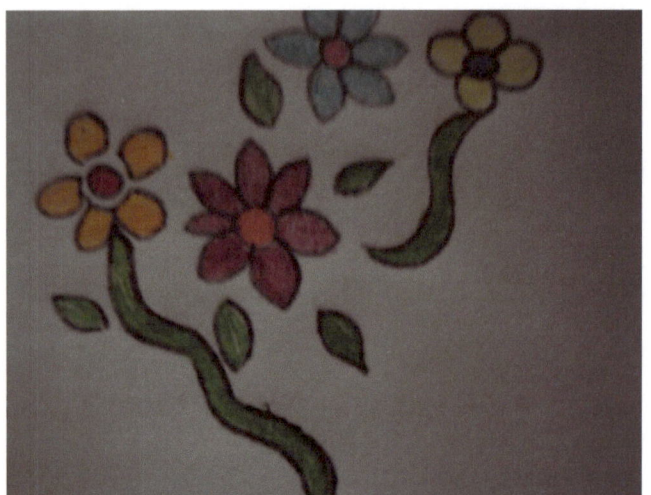

About the Authors

Michael R. Basso has significant experience as a leader in quality and reliability engineering and management in industry, as well as being a college level educator in psychology at Yale University and the University of Connecticut. His experience also includes being a consultant, researcher, and newspaper columnist. Michael is the president of the Connecticut Holistic Health Association.

Dr. Basso has a Ph.D. in professional psychology and biomedical systems, an MS in engineering science, and an MBA with a focus in executive leadership and an interdisciplinary Professional Development Diploma in pathophysiology, neural systems, and education. He also holds a BS in electrical engineering. Michael is certified in quality and reliability engineering and quality auditing, as well as a variety of health related areas.

Dorothy lives in New York with Frankie who has Down Syndrome. She has a daughter, Sandra, another son, Mark, and four grandchildren. Dorothy earned an Associates Degree at the Latin-American Institute in Manhattan and her paralegal certificate at Manhattanville College. She now works as a legal secretary/paralegal for a law firm in Greenwich, CT.

Dorothy was a literacy volunteer for many years starting when her children were in elementary school. She has continued to volunteer to teach English to the new wave of immigrants in her native village, Port Chester, NY. She also has been a member of the parish counsel of her church helping to establish goals for the parish. Presently, she is on a committee at her church which reaches out to the elderly. She was also a member of the Board of Directors of Don Bosco Community Center in Port Chester, NY.

Dorothy is also on the Board of Directors of the Tamarack Tower Foundation in Port Chester, NY as well as corresponding secretary for the TTF. She is also on the Board of Directors of the South East Consortium for Special Services, Inc., located in Mamaroneck, NY.

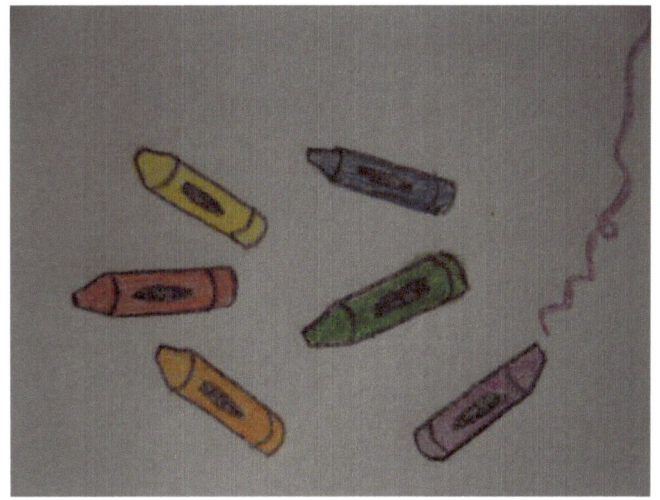

Grandma, I can't wait to see my new baby sister. She was born in the house but the lady who helped Claire be born said that I couldn't see her for a few days.

Here she comes, Bobby!

Hi Claire!!! I am your big brother Bobby…

Mom, she's sooooo cute with her little pink pajamas and booties…but Dad you're not Asian and neither is mom. How come Claire looks like Lee from school? They both have slanty eyes.

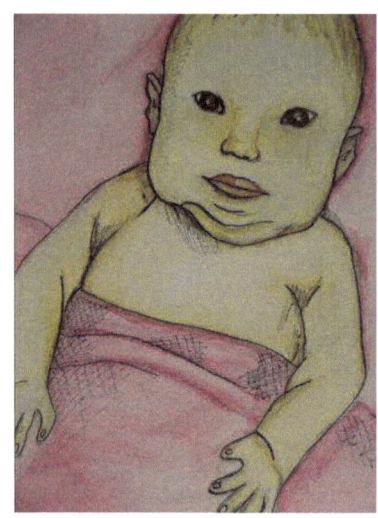

Well Bobby, they sometimes call mentally challenged children a big word called 'mon go loid.'

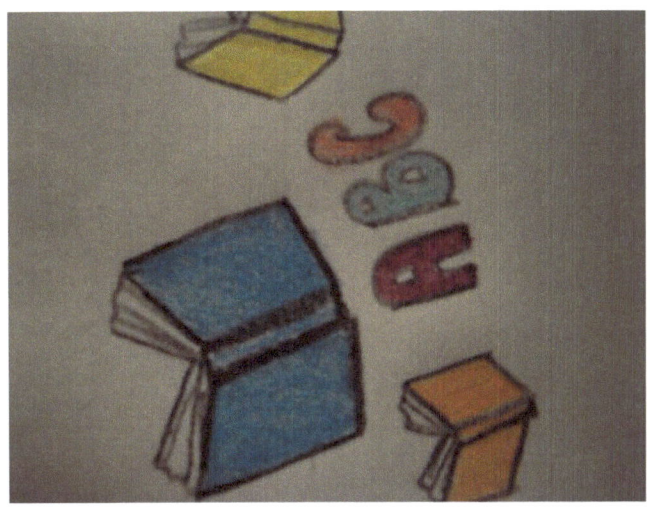

They call them Mongoloid because Asian people, like those from China…also have slanty eyes and their faces sometimes look very similar. Those people are sometimes called mongoloid.

Bobby, it's very important that you realize that because Asian people may look like mentally challenged children that that doesn't mean that they are mentally challenged like Claire. Many Asian people are so smart that they are sometimes called "super stars."

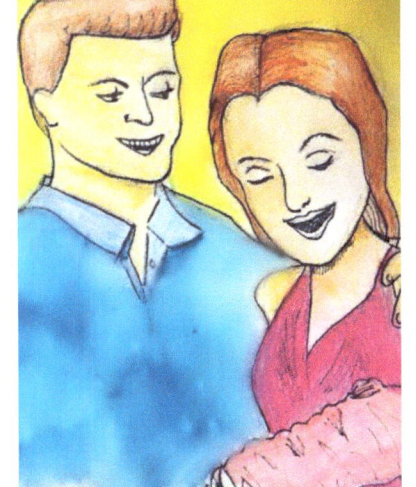

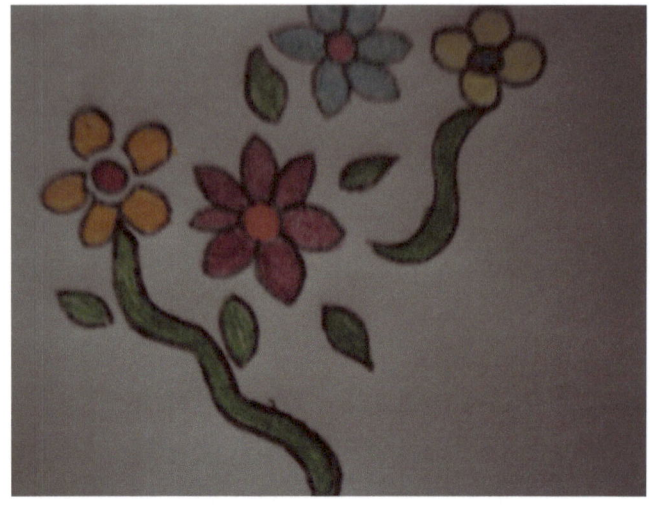

Mom, you're a teacher. What was dad talking about? Aren't mentally challenged kids smart too? And how come Asian people are so smart?

Mentally challenged kids may be very smart in many ways. But they often have to work harder than other kids because their brain is different than other children.

Some mentally challenged children can even play instruments and do sports. I know of one mentally challenged man who learned to play two instruments, he knows how to use a computer and he is even a famous karate expert. Most 'normal' people can't do those things.

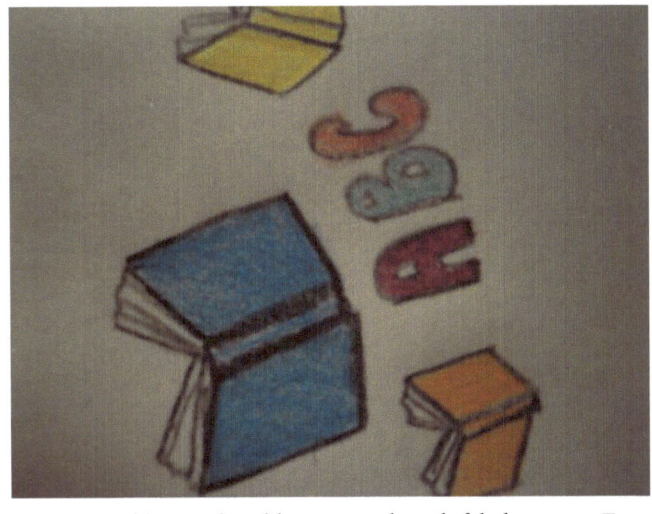

Why was this boy so special, Mom?

Well, Bobby, his mom and dad cared a lot about him. They were told to put him in a special place for mentally challenged children. Instead, he was given special lessons from very patient teachers, who also helped to teach his mom and dad how to be special parents.

Hi, Nana, what are you doing here?

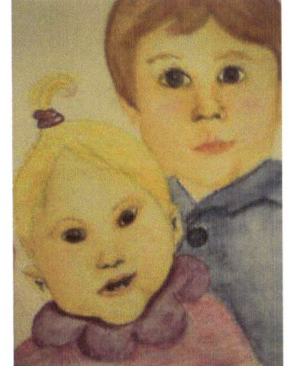

Bobby, your parents asked me to watch Claire. They are going to the library to learn as much as they can about mentally challenged kids and about other places where they can learn even more about being a special parent.

Wait !! Mom, Dad. I want to go to the library too.

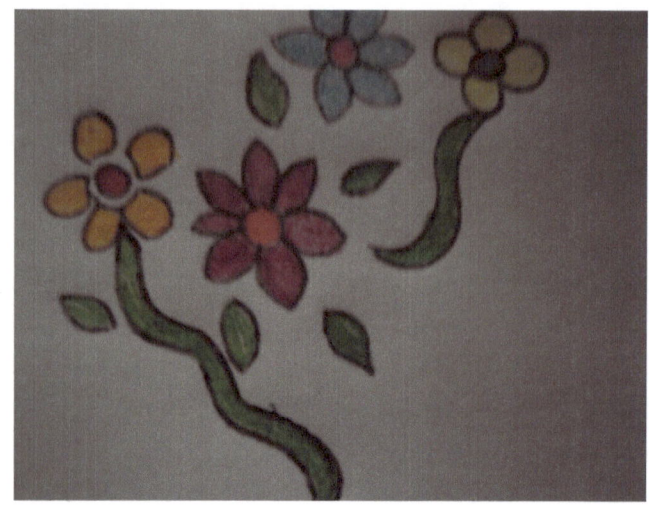

OK, Bobby. Please hurry!

What did you find, Mom?

Bobby, this blue book says that mentally challenged kids have different genes than other kids.

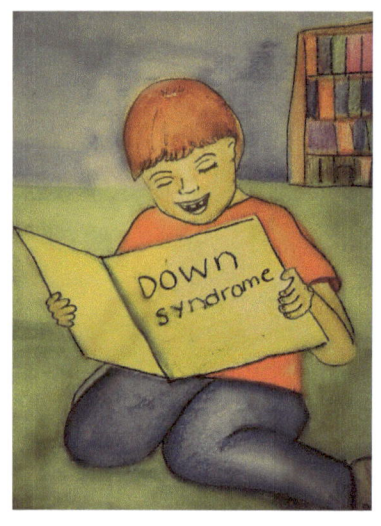

Huh, you mean that they wear different pants! What!

No silly. Genes are like tiny computers that tell our bodies and minds what to do.

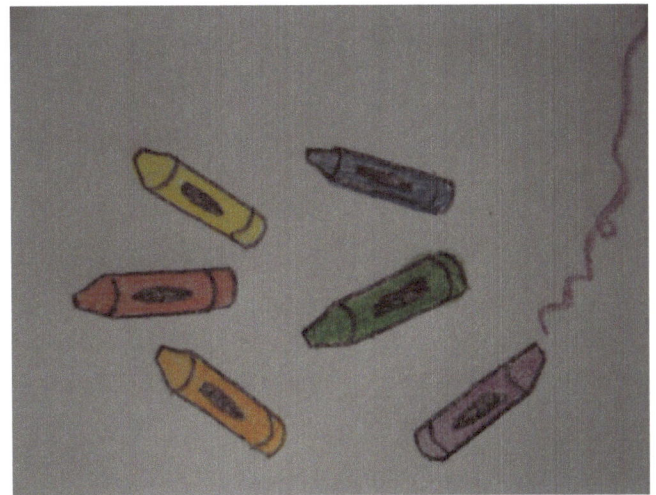

They are present on chromosomes, where lots of genes are in special places. Many mentally challenged children are born with different genes that can make them be less intelligent than other kids.

Says here that some kids are mildly mentally challenged, other kids are severely mentally challenged and still others are somewhere in between. Mildly mentally challenged kids are almost like other children. Some kids are so mentally challenged that they can hardly do much of anything.

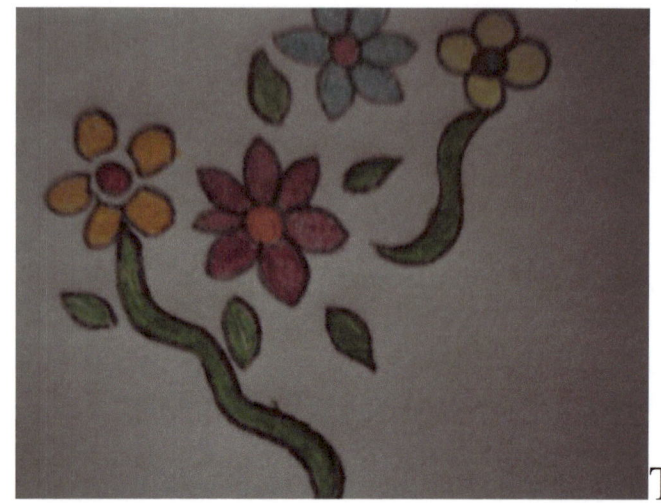This other book says that mentally challenged kids often have other things that are different. Some children have trouble speaking, others may be on the short side, and still others may have faces that are different than other kids.

What's that, Dad?

Bobby, this book's about what may happen when Down Syndrome kids grow up and get older. Says here that many of them get Alzheimer's disease – that's a disease where older people may forget things, and get very confused.

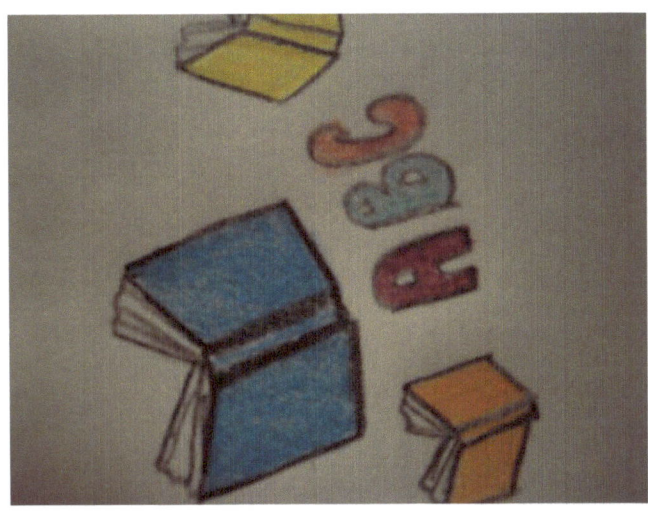

Wow look at this, Bobby. This book tells us that mentally challenged children often have heart defects, but rarely get heart attacks when they get older – so they may be stronger than other kids in some ways. I'll be darned.

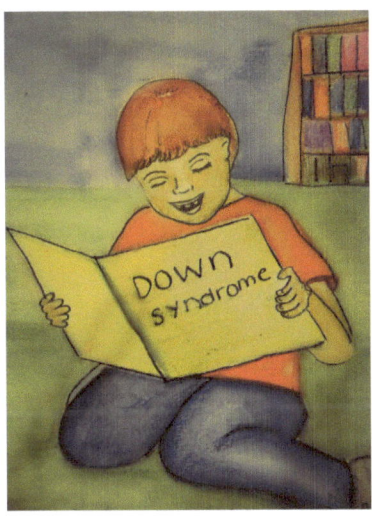

Look here, Burt. This book has lots of places where we can take Claire, like that Southeast Center. Kids learn lots of

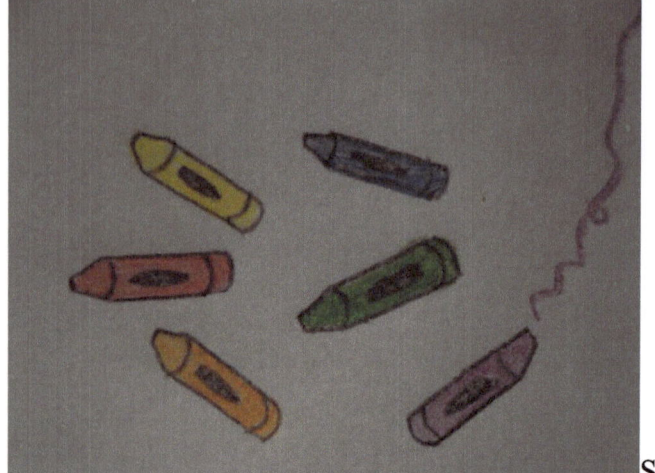

skills in places like that and they can talk to and play with other mentally challenged kids. They have contests, parties and play lots of fun games. It also has lots of places where we can learn more on the computer.

That's great Jane.

Time passed and Claire learned lots of things with the help of her mom and dad…their moms and dads and Bobby too.

Hey mom, what are you doing now?

Bobby, Claire is in kindergarten now and her teachers want us to label things around the house so Claire can learn faster…

That's fun Mom…I'll help you too.

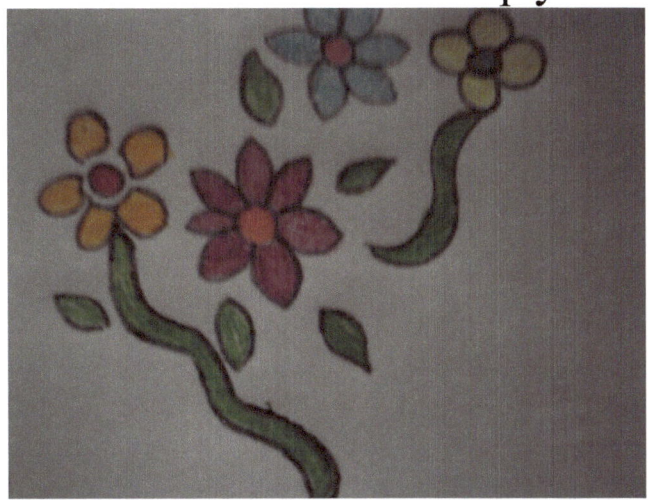

That's great, Mom. I was starting to feel left out….with you and dad paying all that attention to her and none to me.

It just seems that way, Bobby. We love you both ~

Hey Dad, How come it takes Claire sooooo long to learn to ride her bike? That doesn't have anything to do with her mind?

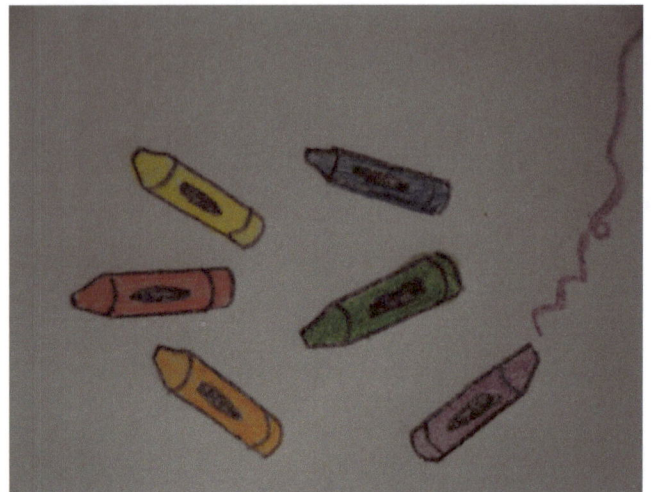

In a way it does, Bobby. The mind has parts that we know about – like when we talk or think…It also has parts that we don't know about that make our hearts beat, help us breathe and even make our muscles work smoothly, like when we ride our bikes.

Down Syndrome kids often have trouble making their muscles work like other kids.

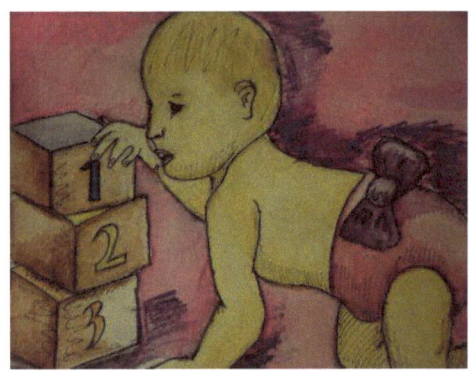

Mom, what are you doing now?

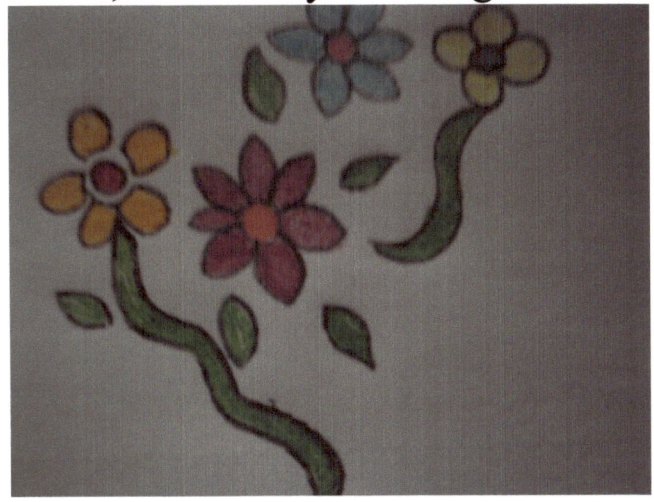

We're labeling objects around the house to make it easier for Claire to read and to talk and to just understand things.

help, Mom?

Wow how cool! Can I

Of course you can, Bobby.

Mom, this is fun and helping makes me like Claire even more. I was starting to get jealous.

I know you were!

Mom, some kid at school has a brother who is mentally challenged, but he can play the xylophone! Can we get a xylophone for Claire and drums for me?

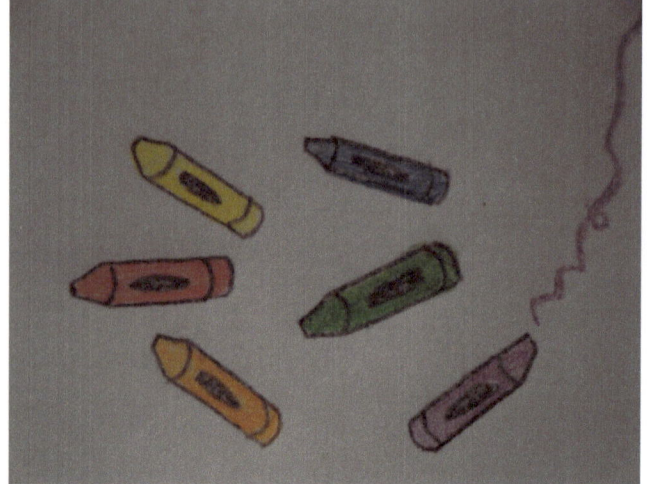

Of course we can.

Wow, Bobby, that will be fun, Claire said.

Claire loved to play the drums and the xylophone too and so did Bobby…..They learned from each other….

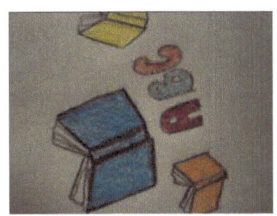

Workbook Section

It's OK for Moms, Dads, Big Sisters, Brothers or others to help you!

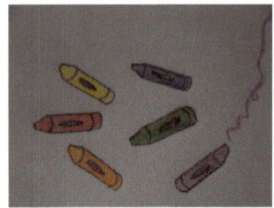

Write down four things that are special about Down Syndrome children?

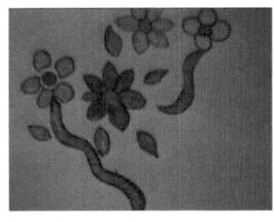 Name one disease that Down Syndrome children commonly get when they get older and one disease that is common among others that mentally challenged people don't usually get.

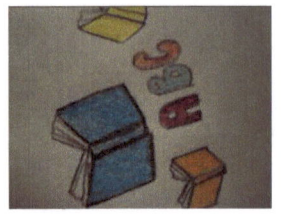 What are some ways that a brother or sister can help their parents deal with a child who is mentally challenged?

1)

2)

3)

4)

5)

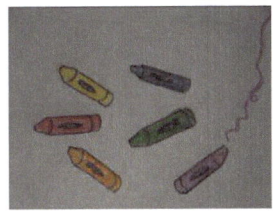 Please think of some major accomplishments that mentally challenged people have accomplished – feel free to ask others, go to the library, check the internet, etc.

1)

2)

3)

4)

5)

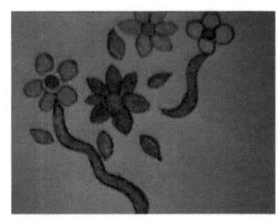 How can families learn more about Down Syndrome?

1)

2)

3)

4)

5)

www.ingramcontent.com/pod-product-compliance
Lightning Source LLC
Chambersburg PA
CBHW060825290526

45792CB00005BB/1796